Simply Tasty V
Cookbo

50+ Easy to Make
Vegetable Recipes F
Lifestyle

ANNIE H

TABLE OF CONTENTS

INTRODUCTION

A large number of individuals who have deliberately inspected creature agribusiness have made plans to go veggie lover. In any case, regardless of whether you choose a veggie lover diet isn't for you, you'll likely leave away from perusing this exposition sold on the advantages of eating what individuals currently call a "plant-based" diet. For what reason am I so sure? Since the motivations to pick an eating routine that is at any rate generally plant-based are overpowering to such an extent that there truly aren't any solid counterarguments. That may clarify why the most unmistakable nourishment governmental issues journalists—including Michael Pollan, Mark Bittman, and Eric Schlosser—advocate an eating routine dependent on plants.

Plant-based weight control plans convey a significant number of the advantages of being vegetarian while requiring just the scarcest exertion. Since you haven't dedicated yourself to being 100 percent anything, there's no motivation to stress that you'll cheat, slip, or mess up. You can follow a plant-based eating routine and still eat Thanksgiving turkey or a late spring grill. In the event that being 100 percent veggie lover is something individuals focus on, being plant-based is more something they incline toward.

Perhaps the best thing about the plant-based idea is that it frequently gets under way an "idealistic cycle," where one positive change prompts another and afterward to another. At the point when you normally attempt new veggie lover nourishments, your top picks will in general consequently become piece of your ordinary eating regimen. So as time passes by, your eating regimen will probably move in a veggie lover heading with no deliberate exertion on your part. A lot of current veggie lovers arrived by bit by bit sliding down the plant-based slant. After some time spent eating expanding measures of plant-based nourishments, they understood that they were only a couple of little and simple advances from turning out to be absolutely vegetarian.

There are various adorable and accommodating neologisms appended to the plant-based camp: reducetarian, flexitarian, chegan, plant-solid, and even veganish. On the off chance that any of these terms impacts you, simply snatch tightly to it and start thinking thusly as you start attempting more veggie lover and vegetarian suppers.

Also, there are a few other related ideas you may discover supportive, including: Meatless Mondays, Mark Bittman's Vegan Before 6:00 arrangement, or taking a completely vegetarian diet out for a 21-day test drive. These conceivable outcomes can move huge change without forcing prerequisites for long lasting flawlessness.

Of the numerous motivations to go plant-based, maybe the best of all is the absence of a reasonable counterargument. In the entirety of my years expounding on nourishment legislative issues, I've not even once observed anybody (other than a couple paleo diet fan) make a genuine endeavor to contend against eating for the most part plants, since the preferences are unquestionable. Handfuls and many examinations show that eating more products of the soil can drastically diminish paces of malignant growth, diabetes, and circulatory malady. Furthermore, obviously, plant-based weight control plans likewise keep livestock from butcher, while all the while securing nature.

BREAKFAST & SMOOTHIES

01. Wild Ginger Green Smoothie

Preparation Time: 5 minutes
Cooking Time: 0 minute
Servings: 1

Ingredients:
- 1/2 cup pineapple chunks, frozen
- 1/2 cup chopped kale
- 1/2 frozen banana
- 1 tablespoon lime juice
- 2 inches ginger, peeled, chopped
- 1/2 cup coconut milk, unsweetened
- 1/2 cup coconut water

Directions:
1. Place all the ingredients in the order in a food processor or blender and then pulse for 2 to 3 minutes at high speed until smooth.
2. Pour the smoothie into a glass and then serve.

Nutrition:
Calories: 331 Cal
Fat: 14 g
Carbs: 40 g
Protein: 16 g
Fiber: 9 g

02. Berry Beet Velvet Smoothie

Preparation Time: 5 minutes
Cooking Time: 0 minute
Servings: 1
Ingredients:

- 1/2 of frozen banana
- 1 cup mixed red berries
- 1 Medjool date, pitted
- 1 small beet, peeled, chopped
- 1 tablespoon cacao powder
- 1 teaspoon chia seeds
- 1/4 teaspoon vanilla extract, unsweetened
- 1/2 teaspoon lemon juice
- 2 teaspoons coconut butter
- 1 cup coconut milk, unsweetened

Directions:

1. Place all the ingredients in the order in a food processor or blender and then pulse for 2 to 3 minutes at high speed until smooth.
2. Pour the smoothie into a glass and then serve.

Nutrition:

Calories: 234 Cal   Protein: 11 g
Fat: 5 g   Fiber: 7 g
Carbs: 42 g

03. **Spiced Strawberry Smoothie**

Preparation Time: 5 minutes
Cooking Time: 0 minute
Servings: 1
Ingredients:

- 1 tablespoon goji berries, soaked
- 1 cup strawberries
- 1/8 teaspoon sea salt
- 1 frozen banana
- 1 Medjool date, pitted
- 1 scoop vanilla-flavored whey protein
- 2 tablespoons lemon juice
- ¼ teaspoon ground ginger
- ½ teaspoon ground cinnamon
- 1 tablespoon almond butter
- 1 cup almond milk, unsweetened

Directions:

1. Place all the ingredients in the order in a food processor or blender and then pulse for 2 to 3 minutes at high speed until smooth.
2. Pour the smoothie into a glass and then serve.

Nutrition:
Calories: 182 Cal
Fat: 1.3 g

Carbs: 34 g
Protein: 6.4 g
Fiber: 0.7 g

04. Banana Bread Shake With Walnut Milk

Preparation Time: 5 minutes
Cooking Time: 0 minute
Servings: 2
Ingredients:

- 2 cups sliced frozen bananas
- 3 cups walnut milk
- 1/8 teaspoon grated nutmeg
- 1 tablespoon maple syrup
- 1 teaspoon ground cinnamon
- 1/2 teaspoon vanilla extract, unsweetened
- 2 tablespoons cacao nibs

Directions:

1. Place all the ingredients in the order in a food processor or blender and then pulse for 2 to 3 minutes at high speed until smooth.
2. Pour the smoothie into two glasses and then serve.

Nutrition:
Calories: 339.8 Cal
Fat: 19 g
Carbs: 39 g

Protein: 4.3 g
Fiber: 1 g

05. Double Chocolate Hazelnut Espresso Shake

Preparation Time: 5 minutes
Cooking Time: 0 minute
Servings: 1
Ingredients:

- 1 frozen banana, sliced
- 1/4 cup roasted hazelnuts
- 4 Medjool dates, pitted, soaked
- 2 tablespoons cacao nibs, unsweetened
- 1 1/2 tablespoons cacao powder, unsweetened
- 1/8 teaspoon sea salt
- 1 teaspoon vanilla extract, unsweetened
- 1 cup almond milk, unsweetened
- 1/2 cup ice
- 4 ounces espresso, chilled

Directions:
1. Place all the ingredients in the order in a food processor or blender and then pulse for 2 to 3 minutes at high speed until smooth.
2. Pour the smoothie into a glass and then serve.

Nutrition:
Calories: 210 Cal
Fat: 5 g
Carbs: 27 g
Protein: 16.8 g
Fiber: 0.2 g

06. Strawberry, Banana And Coconut Shake

Preparation Time: 5 minutes
Cooking Time: 0 minute
Servings: 1
Ingredients:

- 1 tablespoon coconut flakes
- 1 1/2 cups frozen banana slices
- 8 strawberries, sliced
- 1/2 cup coconut milk, unsweetened
- 1/4 cup strawberries for topping

Directions:

1. Place all the ingredients in the order in a food processor or blender, except for topping and then pulse for 2 to 3 minutes at high speed until smooth.
2. Pour the smoothie into a glass and then serve.

Nutrition:
Calories: 335 Cal
Fat: 5 g
Carbs: 75 g
Protein: 4 g
Fiber: 9 g

07. Tropical Vibes Green Smoothie

Preparation Time: 5 minutes
Cooking Time: 0 minute
Servings: 1
Ingredients:

- 2 stalks of kale, ripped
- 1 frozen banana
- 1 mango, peeled, pitted, chopped
- 1/8 teaspoon sea salt
- ¼ cup of coconut yogurt
- ½ teaspoon vanilla extract, unsweetened
- 1 tablespoon ginger juice
- ½ cup of orange juice
- ½ cup of coconut water

Directions:

1. Place all the ingredients in the order in a food processor or blender and then pulse for 2 to 3 minutes at high speed until smooth.
2. Pour the smoothie into a glass and then serve.

Nutrition:

Calories: 197.5 Cal
Fat: 1.3 g
Carbs: 30 g

Protein: 16.3 g
Fiber: 4.8 g

08. Peanut Butter And Mocha Smoothie

Preparation Time: 5 minutes
Cooking Time: 0 minute
Servings: 1
Ingredients:

- 1 frozen banana, chopped
- 1 scoop of chocolate protein powder
- 2 tablespoons rolled oats
- 1/8 teaspoon sea salt
- ¼ teaspoon vanilla extract, unsweetened
- 1 teaspoon cocoa powder, unsweetened
- 2 tablespoons peanut butter
- 1 shot of espresso
- ½ cup almond milk, unsweetened

Directions:
1. Place all the ingredients in the order in a food processor or blender and then pulse for 2 to 3 minutes at high speed until smooth.
2. Pour the smoothie into a glass and then serve.

Nutrition:

Calories: 380 Cal   Protein: 38 g
Fat: 14 g   Fiber: 4 g
Carbs: 29 g

09. Tahini Shake With Cinnamon And Lime

Preparation Time: 5 minutes
Cooking Time: 0 minute
Servings: 1
Ingredients:

- 1 frozen banana
- 2 tablespoons tahini
- 1/8 teaspoon sea salt
- ¾ teaspoon ground cinnamon
- ¼ teaspoon vanilla extract, unsweetened
- 2 teaspoons lime juice
- 1 cup almond milk, unsweetened

Directions:

1. Place all the ingredients in the order in a food processor or blender and then pulse for 2 to 3 minutes at high speed until smooth.
2. Pour the smoothie into a glass and then serve.

Nutrition:
Calories: 225 Cal
Fat: 15 g
Carbs: 22 g
Protein: 6 g
Fiber: 8 g

10. Ginger And Greens Smoothie

Preparation Time: 5 minutes
Cooking Time: 0 minute
Servings: 1
Ingredients:

- 1 frozen banana
- 2 cups baby spinach
- 2-inch piece of ginger, peeled, chopped
- ¼ teaspoon cinnamon
- ¼ teaspoon vanilla extract, unsweetened
- 1/8 teaspoon salt
- 1 scoop vanilla protein powder
- 1/8 teaspoon cayenne pepper
- 2 tablespoons lemon juice
- 1 cup of orange juice

Directions:

1. Place all the ingredients in the order in a food processor or blender and then pulse for 2 to 3 minutes at high speed until smooth.
2. Pour the smoothie into a glass and then serve.

Nutrition:

Calories: 320 Cal   Protein: 10 g
Fat: 7 g   Fiber: 12
Carbs: 64 g

11. Peanut Butter-Banana Green Smoothie

Ingredients:

- 1 cup unsweetened almond milk
- 2 cups of spinach, chopped
- 2 frozen ripe bananas
- 1 tbsp. peanut butter
- 2 ice cubes

Directions:

Place all ingredients in a blender and blend until smooth.

12. Raspberry Mango Green Smoothie

Ingredients:

- 3 cups fresh spinach
- 1 ripe banana, frozen
- 1 cup soy milk
- 1/2 cup mango, diced
- 1/3 cup fresh raspberries

Directions:

Blend all ingredients in a blender until smooth. Serve in cups.

13. Pineapple Orange Green Smoothie

Ingredients:

- 1 banana
- 1/3 cup kale, chopped
- 1/2 cup frozen banana
- 1 tablespoon pineapple
- 1/3 cup orange juice
- 1 tablespoon chia seeds

Directions:
Blend all ingredients in a blender until smooth.

14. Blueberry Green Smoothie

Ingredients:

- 1 tablespoon flax seeds
- 1 cup blueberries
- 1 frozen ripe banana, quartered
- 1/3 cup water, or more to taste
- 3 ice cubes
- 2 leaves kale

Directions:

Blend all ingredients in a blender until smooth. If you would like a thinner smoothie add water.

15. Strawberry Green Smoothie

Ingredients:

- 2 cups coconut water
- 1 cup spinach
- 1 banana
- 6 sliced fresh strawberries

Directions:

Blend coconut water, spinach, banana and strawberries together in a blender until smooth.

MAINS

01. Herbed Mushrooms

Preparation time: 10 minutes
Cooking time: 12 minutes
Servings: 3
Ingredients:

- 10 oyster mushrooms, stems removed
- 1 tablespoon mixed oregano and basil dried
- 1 tablespoon cashew cheese, grated
- A drizzle of olive oil
- 1 tablespoon dill, chopped
- Salt and black pepper to the taste

Directions:

1. Season mushrooms with salt, pepper, mixed herbs, drizzle the oil over them, place them in your air fryer and Cooking Time: at 360 degrees F for 6 minutes.
2. Add cashew cheese and dill, Cooking Time: for 6 minutes more, divide between plates and serve.
3. Enjoy!

Nutrition: calories 210, fat 7, fiber 1, carbs 12, protein 6

02. Corn With Tofu

Preparation time: 10 minutes
Cooking time: 15 minutes
Servings: 4
Ingredients:

- 4 cups corn
- Salt and black pepper to the taste
- 1 tablespoon olive oil
- Juice of 2 limes
- 2 teaspoon smoked paprika
- ½ cup soft tofu, crumbled

Directions:

1. In your air fryer, mix oil with corn, salt, pepper, lime juice and paprika, toss well, cover and Cooking Time: at 400 degrees F for 15 minutes.
2. Divide between plates, sprinkle tofu crumbles all over and serve hot.
3. Enjoy!

Nutrition: calories 160, fat 2, fiber 2, carbs 12, protein 4

03. Garlicky Potatoes

Preparation time: 10 minutes
Cooking time: 40 minutes
Servings: 3
Ingredients:

- 3 big potatoes, peeled and cut into wedges
- Salt and black pepper to the taste
- 2 tablespoons olive oil
- 1 teaspoons sweet paprika
- 2 tablespoons garlic, minced
- 1 tablespoon parsley, chopped

Directions:

1. Put the potatoes in your air fryer's basket, add salt, pepper, garlic, parsley, paprika and oil, toss to coat and Cooking Time: at 392 degrees F for 40 minutes.
2. Divide them between plates and serve hot.
3. Enjoy!

Nutrition: calories 123, fat 1, fiber 2, carbs 21, protein 3

04. Tasty Veggie Mix

Preparation time: 10 minutes
Cooking time: 15 minutes
Servings: 4
Ingredients:

- 2 red onions, cut into chunks
- 2 zucchinis, cut into medium chunks
- 3 tomatoes, cut into wedges
- ¼ cup black olives, pitted and cut into halves
- ¼ cup olive oil
- Salt and black pepper to the taste
- 1 garlic clove, minced
- 1 tablespoon mustard
- 1 tablespoon lemon juice
- ½ cup parsley, chopped

Directions:

1. In your air fryer's pan, mix onion with zucchini, olives, tomatoes, salt, pepper, oil, garlic, mustard and lemon juice, toss, cover and Cooking Time: at 370 degrees F for 15 minutes.
2. Add parsley, toss, divide between plates and serve.
3. Enjoy!

Nutrition:

calories 210,

fat 1,

fiber 4,

carbs 7,

protein 11

05. French Mushroom Mix

Preparation time: 10 minutes
Cooking time: 25 minutes
Servings: 4
Ingredients:

- 2 pounds mushrooms, halved
- 2 teaspoons herbs de Provence
- ½ teaspoon garlic powder
- 1 tablespoon olive oil

Directions:
1. Heat up a pan with the oil over medium heat, add herbs and heat them up for 2 minutes.
2. Add mushrooms and garlic powder, stir, introduce pan in your air fryer's basket and Cooking Time: at 360 degrees F for 25 minutes.
3. Divide between plates and serve.
4. Enjoy!

Nutrition: calories 152, fat 2, fiber 4, carbs 9, protein 7

06. Easy Broccoli Mix

Preparation time: 10 minutes
Cooking time: 20 minutes
Servings: 4
Ingredients:

- 2 broccoli heads, florets separated
- Juice of ½ lemon
- 1 tablespoon olive oil
- 2 teaspoons sweet paprika
- Salt and black pepper to the taste
- 3 garlic cloves, minced
- 1 tablespoon sesame seeds

Directions:

1. In a bowl, mix broccoli with lemon juice, olive oil, paprika, salt, pepper and garlic, toss to coat, transfer to your air fryer's basket, Cooking Time: at 360 degrees G for 15 minutes, sprinkle sesame seeds, Cooking Time: for 5 minutes more and divide between plates.
2. Serve right away.
3. Enjoy!

Nutrition: calories 156, fat 4, fiber 3, carbs 12, protein 5

07. Zucchini And Squash Salad

Preparation time: 10 minutes
Cooking time: 25 minutes
Servings: 4
Ingredients:

- 6 teaspoons olive oil
- 1 pound zucchinis, cut into half moons
- ½ pound carrots, cubed
- 1 yellow squash, cut into chunks
- Salt and white pepper to the taste
- 1 tablespoon tarragon, chopped
- 2 tablespoons tomato paste

Directions:
1. In your air fryer's pan, mix oil with zucchinis, carrots, squash, salt, pepper, tarragon and tomato paste, cover and Cooking Time: at 400 degrees F for 25 minutes.
2. Divide between plates and serve.
3. Enjoy!

Nutrition: calories 170, fat 2, fiber 2, carbs 12, protein 5

08. Indian Cauliflower Mix

Preparation time: 10 minutes
Cooking time: 20 minutes
Servings: 4
Ingredients:

- 3 cups cauliflower florets
- Salt and black pepper to the taste
- A drizzle of olive oil
- ½ cup veggie stock
- ¼ teaspoon turmeric powder
- 1 and ½ teaspoon red chili powder
- 1 tablespoon ginger paste
- 2 teaspoons lemon juice
- 2 tablespoons water

Directions:

1. In your air fryer's pan, mix stock with cauliflower, oil, salt, pepper, turmeric, chili powder, ginger paste, lemon juice and water, stir, cover and Cooking Time: at 400 degrees F for 10 minutes and at 360 degrees F for another 10 minutes.
2. Divide between bowls and serve.
3. Enjoy!

Nutrition: calories 150, fat 1, fiber 2, carbs 12, protein 3

09. "Baked" Potatoes

Preparation time: 10 minutes
Cooking time: 40 minutes
Servings: 3
Ingredients:

- 3 big baking potatoes
- 1 teaspoon dill, chopped
- 1 tablespoon garlic, minced
- Salt and black pepper to the taste
- 2 tablespoons olive oil

Directions:

1. Prick potatoes with a fork, season with salt and pepper to the taste, rub with the oil, garlic and dill, place them in your air fryer's basket and Cooking Time: at 392 degrees F for 40 minutes.
2. Divide them between plates and serve.
3. Enjoy!

Nutrition: calories 130, fat 2, fiber 3, carbs 23, protein 4

10. Squash Stew

Preparation time: 10 minutes
Cooking time: 30 minutes
Servings: 8

Ingredients:

- 2 carrots, chopped
- 1 yellow onion, chopped
- 2 celery stalks, chopped
- 2 green apples, cored, peeled and chopped
- 4 garlic cloves, minced
- 2 cups butternut squash, peeled and cubed
- 6 ounces canned chickpeas, drained
- 6 ounces canned black beans, drained
- 7 ounces canned coconut milk
- 2 teaspoons chili powder
- 1 teaspoon oregano, dried
- 1 tablespoon cumin, ground
- 2 cups veggie stock
- 2 tablespoons tomato paste
- Salt and black pepper to the taste
- 1 tablespoon cilantro, chopped

Directions:

1. In your air fryer, mix carrots with onion, celery, apples, garlic, squash, chickpeas, black beans, coconut milk, chili powder, oregano, cumin, stock, tomato paste, salt and pepper, stir, cover and Cooking Time: at 370 degrees F for 30 minutes
2. Add cilantro, stir, divide into bowls and serve hot.
3. Enjoy!

Nutrition: calories 332, fat 6, fiber 8, carbs 12, protein 6

10. Squash Stew Servings: 4

Ingredients:

For the mushrooms:

- 1/4 cup olive oil
- 3 tbsp balsamic vinegar
- 3 tbsp low sodium tamari or nama shoyu
- 3 tbsp maple syrup
- Sprinkle pepper
- 4 portobello mushroom tops, cleaned
- Submerge 4 Portobello tops in the marinade. 1 hour will be sufficient for them to be prepared, however medium-term in the refrigerator is far and away superior.

For the Cauliflower Mashed Potatoes:

- 1 cups cashews, crude
- 4 cups cauliflower, slashed into little florets and pieces
- 2 tbsp smooth white miso
- 3 tbsp dietary yeast
- 2 tbsp lemon juice
- Ocean salt and dark pepper to taste
- 1/3 cup (or lesswater

Strategy

1. Place cashews into the bowl of your

nourishment processor, and procedure into a fine powder.

2. Add the miso, lemon juice, healthful yeast, pepper and cauliflower. Heartbeat to join. With the engine of the machine running, include water in a flimsy streamin., until the blend starts to take on a smooth, whipped surface. You may need to stop every now and again to clean the sides of the bowl and help it along.

3. When the blend looks like pureed potatoes, stop, scoop, and serve close by a Portobello top.

12. Quinoa Enchiladas

Adjusted from a formula in Food52

Servings: 6

Ingredients:

- 1 tbsp coconut oil
- 2 cloves garlic, minced
- 1 little yellow onion, cleaved
- 3/4 pounds infant bella mushrooms, hacked
- 1/2 cup diced green bean stews
- 1/2 teaspoon ground cumin
- 1/4 teaspoon ocean salt (or to taste
- 1 can natural, low sodium dark beans or 1/2 cup cooked dark beans
- 1/2 cup cooked quinoa
- 10 6-inch corn tortillas
- 1/4 cup natural, low sodium tomato or enchilada sauce

Technique

1. Preheat broiler to 350 degrees.
2. In an enormous pot over medium warmth, heat coconut oil. Sautee onion and garlic till onion is translucent (around 5-8 min). Include mushrooms and Cooking Time: until fluid has been discharged and vanished (another 5 min).
3. Add the bean stews to the pot and give them a

mix for 2 minutes. Include the cumin, ocean salt, dark beans and quinoa, and keep warming the blend until it's totally warm.

4. Spread a flimsy layer (1/2 cupof marinara or enchilada sauce in the base of a goulash dish. Spot 33% of a cup of quinoa blend in the focal point of a corn tortilla and move it up. Spot the tortilla, crease down, in the goulash dish. Rehash with every outstanding tortilla and afterward spread them with 3/4 cup of extra sauce. Heat for 25 minutes, and serve.

13. Greek Okra And Eggplant Stew

Preparation time: 10 minutes

Cooking time: 25 minutes

Servings: 10

Ingredients:

- 2 cups eggplant, cubed
- 1 butternut squash, peeled and cubed
- 2 cups zucchini, cubed
- 10 ounces tomato sauce
- 1 carrot, sliced
- 1 yellow onion, chopped
- ½ cup veggie stock
- 10 ounces okra
- 1/3 cup raisins
- 2 garlic cloves, minced
- ½ teaspoon turmeric powder
- ½ teaspoon cumin, ground
- ½ teaspoon red pepper flakes, crushed
- ¼ teaspoon sweet paprika
- ¼ teaspoon cinnamon powder

Directions:

1. In your air fryer, mix eggplant with squash, zucchini, tomato sauce, carrot, onion, okra, garlic, stock, raisins, turmeric, cumin, pepper flakes, paprika and cinnamon, stir, cover and Cooking Time: at 360 degrees F for 25 minutes.
2. Divide into bowls and serve.
3. Enjoy!

Nutrition: calories 260, fat 3, fiber 4, carbs 24, protein 3

14. Indian Chickpeas

Preparation time: 10 minutes

Cooking time: 25 minutes

Servings: 14

Ingredients:

- 6 cups canned chickpeas, drained
- 1 cup veggie stock
- 1 yellow onion, chopped
- 1 tablespoon ginger, grated
- 20 garlic cloves, minced
- 8 Thai peppers, chopped
- 2 tablespoons cumin, ground
- 2 tablespoons coriander, ground
- 1 tablespoons red chili powder
- 2 tablespoons garam masala
- 2 tablespoons vegan tamarind paste
- Juice of ½ lemon

Directions:

1. In your air fryer, mix chickpeas with stock, onion ginger, garlic, Thai peppers, cumin, coriander, chili powder, garam masala,

tamarind paste and lemon juice, toss, cover and Cooking Time: at 365 degrees F for 25 minutes.

2. Divide between plates and serve hot.

3. Enjoy!

Nutrition: calories 255, fat 5, fiber 14, carbs 16, protein 17

15. White Beans Stew

Preparation time: 10 minutes
Cooking time: 20 minutes
Servings: 10

Ingredients:

- 2 pounds white beans, cooked
- 3 celery stalks, chopped
- 2 carrots, chopped
- 1 bay leaf
- 1 yellow onion, chopped
- 3 garlic cloves, minced
- 1 teaspoon rosemary, dried
- 1 teaspoon oregano, dried
- 1 teaspoon thyme, dried
- A drizzle of olive oil
- Salt and black pepper to the taste
- 28 ounces canned tomatoes, chopped
- 6 cups chard, chopped

Directions:

1. In your air fryer's pan, mix white beans with celery, carrots, bay leaf, onion, garlic, rosemary, oregano, thyme, oil, salt, pepper, tomatoes and chard, toss, cover and Cooking Time: at 365 degrees F for 20 minutes.
2. Divide into bowls and serve.
3. Enjoy!

Nutrition: calories 341, fat 8, fiber 12, carbs 20, protein 6

SOUPS AND STEWS

01. Chilled Lemongrass And Avocado Soup

Preparation Time: 5 minutes
Cooking Time: 5 minutes + 1 hour refrigeration
Serving Size: 4
Ingredients:

- 2 stalks lemongrass, chopped
- 2 cups chopped avocado pulp
- 2 cups vegetable broth
- 2 lemons, juiced
- 3 tbsp chopped mint leaves + extra to garnish
- Salt and freshly ground black pepper to taste
- 2 cups heavy cream

Directions:

1. In a large pot, add lemongrass, avocado, and vegetable broth; bring to a slow boil over low heat until lemongrass softens and avocado warms through, 5 minutes.
2. Stir in lemon juice, mint leaves, salt, black pepper, and puree ingredients with an immersion blender.
3. Stir in heavy cream and turn heat off.
4. Dish soup into serving bowls, chill for 1 hour, and garnish with some mint leaves. Serve.

Nutrition:

Calories 339, Total Fat 33.3g, Total Carbs 6.58g, Fiber 3g, Net Carbs 3.58g, Protein 3.59g

02. Spinach Soup With Basil

Preparation time: 10 minutes
Cooking time: 5hrs. 5 minutes
Total time: 5 hrs. 15 minutes
Servings: 06

Ingredients:
- 8 ounces potatoes, diced
- 1 medium onion, chopped
- 1 large clove of garlic, chopped
- 1 teaspoon powdered mustard
- 3 cups water
- ¼ teaspoon salt
- Ground cayenne pepper
- ½ cup packed fresh dill
- 10 ounces frozen spinach

How to Prepare:
1. In a low cooker, add olive oil and onion.
2. Sauté for 5 minutes then toss in rest of the soup ingredients.
3. Put on the slow cooker's lid and Cooking Time: for 5 hours on low heat.
4. Once done, puree the soup with a hand blender.
5. Serve warm.

Nutritional Values:
Calories 162
Total Fat 4 g
Saturated Fat 1.9 g
Cholesterol 25 mg
Sodium 101 mg
Total Carbs 17.8 g
Sugar 2.1 g
Fiber 6 g
Protein 4 g

03. Beans With Garam Masala Broth

Preparation Time: 40 minutes
Servings: 2

Ingredients
- Red lentils: 1 cups
- Tomatoes: 1 cup can diced
- Beans: 1 cup can rinsed and drained
- Garam masala: 1 tbsp
- Vegetable oil: 2 tbsp
- Onion: 1 cup chopped
- Garlic: 3 cloves minced
- Ground cumin: 2 tbsp
- Smoked paprika: 1 tsp
- Celery: 1 cup chopped
- Sea salt: 1 tsp
- Lime juice and zest: 3 tbsp
- Fresh cilantro: 3 tbsp chopped
- Water: 2 cups

Directions:
1. Take a large pot and add oil to it
2. On the medium flame, add garlic, celery and onion
3. Add salt, garam masala, and cumin to them and

stir for 5 minutes till they turn brown

4. Add water, lentils, and tomatoes with the juice and bring to boil
5. Bring to boil and heat for 25-30 minutes on low flame
6. Add in lime juice and zest and beans of your choice and stir
7. Serve with cilantro on top

Nutrition:
Carbs: 51.5 g
Protein: 19.1 g
Fats: 15.3 g
Calories: 420 Kcal

04. Chickpeas Puree Pumpkin Soup

Preparation Time: 40 minutes
Servings: 4

Ingredients

- Chickpeas: 2 cups can rinsed and drained
- Pumpkin puree: 1 cup can unsweetened
- Onion: 1 cup finely chopped
- Tomatoes: 1 cup can diced not drained
- Water: 3 cups
- Olive oil: 2 tbsp
- Ground cumin: 1 tbsp
- Garlic powder: 2 tsp
- Chili powder: 1 tsp
- Dried oregano: 2 tsp
- Fresh cilantro: 2 tbsp chopped
- Fine sea salt: 1 tsp
- Fresh lime juice: 2 tbsp

Directions:
1. Take a food processor and add tomatoes and chickpeas and make their puree and set aside
2. Take a large saucepan and add oil on the medium heat
3. Add onion and sauté till it turns brown

4. Add chili powder, cumin, garlic powder, salt, and oregano and stir for a minute
5. Add in the pumpkin, chickpeas puree, and water and mix well
6. Lower the heat and simmer uncover for 25-30 minutes and stir after regular intervals
7. When ready, serve with lime juice and season with salt, pepper, and add cilantro on the top

Nutrition:
Carbs: 30.8g
Protein: 9.25g
Fats: 9.4g

05. Hearty Chili

Preparation Time: 10 Minutes
Cooking Time: 15 Minutes
Servings: 4

Ingredients

- 1 onion, diced
- 2 to 3 garlic cloves, minced
- 1 teaspoon olive oil, or 1 to 2 tablespoons water, vegetable broth, or red wine
- 1 (28-ouncecan tomatoes
- ¼ cup tomato paste, or crushed tomatoes
- 1 (14-ouncecan kidney beans, rinsed and drained, or 1½ cups cooked
- 2 to 3 teaspoons chili powder
- ¼ teaspoon sea salt
- ¼ cup fresh cilantro, or parsley leaves

Directions

1. Preparing the Ingredients.
2. In a large pot, sauté the onion and garlic in the oil, about 5 minutes. Once they're soft, add the tomatoes, tomato paste, beans, and chili powder. Season with the salt.
3. Let simmer for at least 10 minutes, or as long as you like. The flavors will get better the

longer it simmers, and it's even better as leftovers.
4. Garnish with cilantro and serve.

Nutrition: Calories: 160; Protein: 8g; Total fat: 3g; Saturated fat: 11g; Carbohydrates: 29g; Fiber: 7g

06. Black Eyed Peas Stew

Serves: **5**

Time: 30 Minutes

Calories: 338

Protein: 21 Grams

Fat: 4 Grams

Carbs: 58 Grams

Ingredients:

- 1 Can Tomatoes, Crushed
- ¼ Teaspoon Cayenne
- 1 Clove Garlic
- 2 Tablespoons Olive Oil
- 1 Onion
- 2 Cans Black Eyed Peas, Drained
- 8 Ounces Okra, Frozen & Thawed
- Sea Salt to Taste

Directions:

1. Start by brown your onion using olive oil, and then add in your garlic and cayenne. Cook for another minute.

2. Mix in all of your remaining ingredients, simmering until your okra becomes soft.

Interesting Facts: Black Eyed peas are infamous for making delicious hummus! They are loaded with 6 grams of protein per serving, and they are easy. You can also use chickpea water as an egg replacement known as aquafaba!

07. White Bean & Spinach Soup

Serves: 4

Time: 25 Minutes

Calories: 218

Protein: 12 Grams

Fat: 3.3 Grams

Carbs: 37.9 Grams

Ingredients:

- 3 Cups Baby Spinach, Cleaned & Trimmed
- 1 Can White Beans (Roughly 14.5 Ounces)
- 3-4 Cups Vegetable Stock, Homemade
- 1 Shallot, Diced Fine
- 1 Clove Garlic, Minced Fine
- 14.5 Ounces Tomatoes, Diced
- 1 Teaspoon Rosemary
- ½ Cup Shell Pasta, Whole Wheat
- 2 Teaspoons Olive Oil
- Red Pepper Flakes to Taste
- Black Pepper to Taste

Directions:

1. Heat olive oil in a saucepan before sautéing your garlic and shallots
2. Add in your rosemary, beans, broth and tomatoes. Season with your red pepper flakes and black pepper.
3. Put your pasta in, cooking for ten minutes, and then add in your spinach. Cook until it's wilted.

Interesting Facts: Spinach is one of the most superb green veggies out there. Each serving is packed with 3 grams of protein and is a highly encouraged component of the plant-based diet.

08. Cabbage & Beet Stew

Serves: 4

Time: 30 Minutes

Calories: 95

Protein: 1 Gram

Fat: 7 Grams

Carbs: 10 Grams

Ingredients:

- 2 Tablespoons Olive Oil
- 3 Cups Vegetable Broth
- 2 Tablespoons Lemon Juice, Fresh
- ½ Teaspoon Garlic Powder
- ½ Cup Carrots, Shredded
- 2 Cups Cabbage, Shredded
- 1 Cup Beets, Shredded
- Dill for Garnish
- ½ Teaspoon Onion Powder
- Sea Salt & Black Pepper to Taste

Directions:

1. Heat oil in a pot, and then sauté your vegetables.
2. Pour your broth in, mixing in your seasoning. Simmer until it's cooked through, and then top with dill.

Interesting Facts: This oil is a main source of dietary fat in a variety of diets. It contains many vitamins and minerals that play a part in reducing the risk of stroke and lowers cholesterol and high blood pressure and can also aid in weight loss. It is best consumed cold, as when it is heated it can lose some of its nutritive properties (although it is still great to cook with – extra virgin is best), many recommend taking a shot of cold oil olive daily! Bonus: if you don't like the taste or texture add a shot to your smoothie.

09. Red Lentil Soup

Serves: 4

Time: 50 Minutes

Calories: 188

Protein: 12.5 Grams

Fat: 1.2 Grams

Carbs: 33.6 Grams

Ingredients:

- 1 Teaspoon Paprika
- 4 Cups Vegetable Stock
- ¼ Cup Onion, Chopped Fine
- 1 Cup Lentil, Red, Washed & Cleaned
- ½ Cup Potato, Peeled & Diced
- Sea Salt & Black Pepper to Taste

Directions:

1. Rinse your lentils under cold water, and then get out a medium pot.
2. Place your red lentils, potatoes, stock, onion and paprika in the pot.
3. Allow it to simmer.

4. Put the lid on loosely, and cook until your lentils are tender. This will take roughly thirty minutes.
5. Add your salt and pepper, put a cup of the soup in the food processor, and then place the blended soup back into the pot.
6. Serve warm.

Interesting Facts: Potatoes are a great starchy source of potassium and protein. They are pretty inexpensive if you are one that is watching their budget. Bonus: Very heart healthy

10. Thai Squash Soup

Serves: 2

Time: 30 Minutes

Calories: 717.3

Protein: 10.3 Grams

Fat: 48.3 Grams

Carbs: 77.4 Grams

Ingredients:

- 1 Teaspoon Curry Powder
- 1 Tablespoon Olive Oil
- 1 Red Onion, Chopped
- 1 Pint Vegetable Stock
- 1 Butter Squash, Chunked
- 1 Can Coconut Milk (Roughly 13.5 Ounces)

Directions:

1. Get out a pan and heat your olive oil. Once it's heated, add in your onion and cook to soften. This should take two to three

minutes. Add your butternut squash, stock to taste, and curry powder.

2. Simmer. The squash should become tender.
3. Stir in your coconut milk, and then blend until smooth.
4. Return it to the pan to warm, and season with salt and pepper before serving.

Interesting Facts: Coconut oil is full of healthy fats that are absorbed easily in the human body. It is a go-to when it comes to Vegan cooking since it is a great substitute for butter and vegetable oils. It can also be used topically, in treating hair and skin. Bonus: Contains fatty acids that aid in weight loss. Double Bonus: Strengthens the immune system.

11. Sesame Bok Choy

Serves: 4

Time: 13 Minutes

Calories: 76

Protein: 4.4 Grams

Fat: 2.7 Grams

Carbs: 9.8 Grams

Ingredients:

- 1 Head Bok Choy
- 1 Teaspoon Canola Oil
- 1/3 Cup Green Onion, Chopped
- 1 Tablespoon Brown Sugar
- 1 ½ Tablespoon Soy Sauce, Light
- 1 Tablespoon Rice Wine
- ½ Teaspoon Ginger, Ground
- 1 Tablespoon Sesame Seeds

Directions:

1. Cut the stems and tops of your bok choy into one inch pieces.
2. Mix together all remaining ingredients in a bowl.
3. Add your bok choy, and top with your dressing.
4. Fry until tender, which should take eight to ten minutes.

Interesting Facts: Sesame seeds can be easily added to crackers, bread, salads, and stir-fry meals. Bonus: Help in lowering cholesterol and high blood pressure. Double bonus: Help with asthma, arthritis, and migraines!

12. Simple Chili

Serves: 4

Time: 30 Minutes

Calories: 160

Protein: 8 Grams

Fat: 3 Grams

Carbs: 29 Grams

Ingredients:

- 1 Onion, Diced
- 1 Teaspoon Olive Oil
- 3 Cloves Garlic, Minced
- 28 Ounces Tomatoes, Canned
- ¼ Cup Tomato Paste
- 14 Ounces Kidney Beans, Canned, Rinsed & Dried
- 2-3 Teaspoons Chili Powder
- ¼ Cup Cilantro, Fresh (or Parsley)
- ¼ Teaspoon Sea Salt, Fine

Directions:

1. Get out a pot, and sauté your onion and garlic in your oil at the bottom cook for five minutes. Add in your tomato paste, tomatoes, beans, and chili powder. Season with salt.
2. Allow it to simmer for ten to twenty minutes.
3. Garnish with cilantro or parsley to serve.

Interesting Facts: Kidney beans are packed with Vitamin B6, potassium, folate, and fiber. Every serving has 7.6 grams of protein. They can easily be used to make yummy veggie burgers, vegan brownies or a killer vegan Mexican meal!

13. Cauliflower Rice Tabbouleh

Serves: 4

Time: 20 Minutes

Calories: 220

Protein: 7 Grams

Fat: 15 Grams

Carbs: 20 Grams

Ingredients:

- 4 Cups Cauliflower Rice
- 1 ½ Cups Cherry Tomatoes, Quartered
- 3-4 Tablespoons Olive Oil
- 1 Cup Parsley, Fresh & Chopped
- 1 Cup Mint, Fresh & Chopped
- 1 Cup Snap Peas, Sliced Thin
- 1 Small Cucumber, Cut into ¼ Inch Pieces
- ¼ Cup Scallions, Sliced Thin
- 3-4 Tablespoons Lemon Juice, Fresh
- 1 Teaspoon Sea Salt, Fine
- ½ Teaspoon Black Pepper

Directions:

1. Get out a bowl and combine your cauliflower rice, tomatoes, mint, parsley, cucumbers, scallions and snap peas together. Toss until combined.
2. Add your olive oil and lemon juice before tossing again. Season with salt and pepper.

Interesting Facts: Cauliflower: This vegetable is an extremely high source of vitamin A, vitamin B1, B2 and B3.

14. Grilled Eggplant Steaks

Serves: 6

Time: 35 Minutes

Calories: 86

Protein: 8 Grams

Fat: 7 Grams

Carbs: 12 Grams

Ingredients:

- 4 Roma Tomatoes, Diced
- 8 Ounces Feta, Diced
- 2 Eggplants
- 1 Tablespoon Olive Oil
- 1 Cup Parsley, Chopped
- 1 Cucumber, Diced
- Sea Salt & Black Pepper to Taste

Directions:

1. Slice your eggplants into three thick steaks, and then drizzle with oil. Season then grill for four minutes per side in a pan.
2. Top with the remaining ingredients.

Interesting Facts: Eggplant has a variety of vital vitamins and minerals within it's compound. It is high in folic acid, vitamin C, manganese and vitamin K. It aids weight lose and cognitive function. Eggplant is a great meat replacement in a lasagna!

15. Ratatouille

Serves: 10

Time: 1 Hour 15 Minutes

Calories: 90

Protein: 3 Grams

Fat: 25 Grams

Carbs: 13 Grams

Ingredients:

- 2 Tablespoons Olive Oil
- 2 Eggplants, Peeled & Cubed
- 8 Zucchini, Chopped
- 4 Tomatoes, Chopped
- ¼ Cup Basil, Chopped
- 4 Thyme Sprigs
- 2 Yellow Onions, Diced
- 3 Cloves Garlic, Minced
- 3 Bell Peppers, Chopped
- 1 Bay Leaf
- Sea Salt to Taste

Directions:

1. Salt your eggplant and leave it in a strainer.
2. Heat a teaspoon of oil in a Dutch oven, cooking your onions for ten minutes. Season with salt.
3. Mix your peppers in, cooking for five more minutes.
4. Place this mixture in a bowl.
5. Heat your oil and sauté zucchini, sprinkling with salt. Cook for five minutes, and place it in the same bowl.
6. Rinse your eggplant, squeezing the water out, and heat another two teaspoons of oil in your Dutch oven. Cook your eggplant for ten minutes, placing it in your vegetable bowl.
7. Heat the remaining oil and cook your garlic. Add in your tomatoes, thyme sprigs and bay leaves to deglaze the bottom.
8. Toss your vegetables back in, and then bring it to a simmer.
9. Simmer for forty-five minutes, and make sure to stir. Discard your thyme and bay leaf. Mix in your basil and serve warm.

Interesting Facts: Eggplant has a variety of vital vitamins and minerals within it's compound. It is high in folic acid, vitamin C, manganese and vitamin K. It aids weight lose and cognitive function. Eggplant is a great meat replacement in a lasagna!

DINNER RECIPES

01. Fried Pineapple Rice

Serves: 6

Time: 30 Minutes

Calories: 179

Protein: 3 Grams

Fat: 4.4 Grams

Carbs: 32.6 Grams

Ingredients:

- 2-3 Cups Brown Rice, Cooked & Cooled
- 1 Tablespoon Sesame Oil
- 2 Tablespoons Raisins (Optional)
- 1 Onion, Small & Chopped
- ½ -3/4 Cup Pineapple, Chopped
- 1 Tablespoon Soy Sauce (Or Braggs Liquid Amino)
- ½ Teaspoon Turmeric
- 1 Tomato, Chopped
- 1 Teaspoon Curry Powder
- 2 Tablespoons Cilantro, Fresh & Chopped
- Sea Salt & Black Pepper to Taste

Directions:

1. Start by getting out a sauce pan, and then add your sesame oil to the pan. Sauté your onions until they turn translucent.
2. Add in your cooked rice, soy sauce, pineapple, curry powder and turmeric.
3. Mix well and cook for eight to ten minutes.
4. Serve with cilantro, and season with salt and pepper.

Interesting Facts: *Pineapple:* This juicy and delicious fruit can be devoured in an array of ways, which means it is a good item to incorporate into meals. Bonus: Since pineapples are full of anti-inflammatory nutrients, they aid in reducing stroke and heart attacks. Double Bonus: Pineapples have also been known to increase fertility!

02. Tomato Gazpacho

Serves: 6

Time: 2 Hours 25 Minutes

Calories: 181

Protein: 3 Grams

Fat: 14 Grams

Carbs: 14 Grams

Ingredients:

- 2 Tablespoons + 1 Teaspoon Red Wine Vinegar, Divided
- ½ Teaspoon Pepper
- 1 Teaspoon Sea Salt
- 1 Avocado,
- ¼ Cup Basil, Fresh & Chopped
- 3 Tablespoons + 2 Teaspoons Olive Oil, Divided
- 1 Clove Garlic, crushed
- 1 Red Bell Pepper, Sliced & Seeded
- 1 Cucumber, Chunked
- 2 ½ lbs. Large Tomatoes, Cored & Chopped

Directions:

1. Place half of your cucumber, bell pepper, and ¼ cup of each tomatoes in a bowl, covering. Set it in the fried.
2. Puree your remaining tomatoes, cucumber and bell pepper with garlic, three tablespoons oil, two tablespoons of vinegar, sea salt and black pepper into a blender, blending until smooth. Transfer it to a bowl, and chill for two hours.
3. Chop the avocado, adding it to your chopped vegetables, adding your remaining oil, vinegar, salt, pepper and basil.
4. Ladle your tomato puree mixture into bowls, and serve with chopped vegetables as a salad.

Interesting Facts: Avocados themselves are ranked within the top five of the healthiest foods on the planet, so you know that the oil that is produced from them is too. It is loaded with healthy fats and essential fatty acids. Like race bran oil it is perfect to cook with as well! Bonus: Helps in the prevention of diabetes and lowers cholesterol levels.

03. Black Bean Burgers

Serves: 6

Time: 25 Minutes

Calories: 173

Protein: 7.3 Grams

Fat: 3.2 Grams

Carbs: 29.7 Grams

Ingredients:

- 1 Onion, Diced
- ½ Cup Corn Nibs
- 2 Cloves Garlic, Minced
- ½ Teaspoon Oregano, Dried
- ½ Cup Flour
- 1 Jalapeno Pepper, Small
- 2 Cups Black Beans, Mashed & Canned
- ¼ Cup Breadcrumbs (Vegan)
- 2 Teaspoons Parsley, Minced
- ¼ Teaspoon Cumin
- 1 Tablespoon Olive Oil

- 2 Teaspoons Chili Powder
- ½ Red Pepper, Diced
- Sea Salt to Taste

Directions:

1. Set your flour on a plate, and then get out your garlic, onion, peppers and oregano, throwing it in a pan. Cook over medium-high heat, and then cook until the onions are translucent. Place the peppers in, and sauté until tender.
2. Cook for two minutes, and then set it to the side.
3. Use a potato masher to mash your black beans, and then stir in the vegetables, cumin, breadcrumbs, parsley, salt and chili powder, and then divide it into six patties.
4. Coat each side, and then cook until it's fried on each side.

Interesting Facts: Potatoes are a great starchy source of potassium and protein. They are pretty inexpensive if you are one that is watching their budget. Bonus: Very heart healthy!

04. Sushi Bowl

Serves: 1

Time: 40 Minutes

Calories: 467

Protein: 22 Grams

Fat: 20 Grams

Carbs: 56 Grams

Ingredients:

- ½ Cup Edamame Beans, Shelled & Fresh
- ¾ Cup Brown Rice, Cooked
- ½ Cup Spinach, Chopped
- ¼ Cup Bell Pepper, Sliced
- ¼ Cup Avocado, Sliced
- ¼ Cup Cilantro, Fresh & Chopped
- 1 Scallion, Chopped
- ¼ Nori Sheet
- 1-2 Tablespoons Tamari
- 1 Tablespoon Sesame Seeds, Optional

Directions:

1. Steam your edamame beans, and then assemble your edamame, rice, avocado, spinach, cilantro, scallions and bell pepper into a bowl.
2. Cut the nori into ribbons, sprinkling it on top, drizzling with tamari and sesame seeds before serving.

Interesting Facts: Avocados are known as miracle fruits in the world of Veganism. They are a true super-fruit and incredibly beneficial. They are one of the best things to eat if you are looking to incorporate more fatty acids in your diet. They are also loaded with 20 various minerals and vitamins. Plus, they are easy to incorporate into dishes all throughout the day!

05. Tofu Poke

Serves: 4

Time: 30 Minutes

Calories: 262

Protein: 16 Grams

Fat: 15 Grams

Carbs: 19 Grams

Ingredients:

- ¾ Cup Scallions, Sliced Thin
- 1 ½ Tablespoons Mirin
- ¼ Cup Tamari
- 1 ½ Tablespoon Dark Sesame Oil, Toasted
- 1 Tablespoon Sesame Seeds, Toasted (Optional)
- 2 Teaspoons Ginger, fresh & Grated
- ½ Teaspoon Red Pepper, crushed
- 12 Ounces Extra Firm Tofu, Drained & Cut into ½ Inch Pieces
- 4 Cups Zucchini Noodles
- 2 Tablespoons Rice Vinegar
- 2 Cups Carrots, Shredded

- 2 Cups Pea Shoots
- ¼ Cup Basil, Fresh & Chopped
- ¼ Cup Peanuts, Toasted & Chopped (Optional)

Directions:

1. Wisk your tamari, mirin, sesame seeds, oil, ginger, red pepper, and scallion greens in a bowl. Set two tablespoons of this sauce aside, and add the tofu to the remaining sauce. Toss to coat.
2. Combine your vinegar and zucchini noodles in a bowl.
3. Divide it between four bowls, topping with tofu, carrots, and a tablespoon of basil and peanuts.
4. Drizzle with sauce before serving.

Interesting Facts: Sesame seeds can be easily added to crackers, bread, salads, and stir-fry meals. Bonus: Help in lowering cholesterol and high blood pressure. Double bonus: Help with asthma, arthritis, and migraines!

CONCLUSION

Thanks for making to the end! I hope you enjoy all the recipes herein. If dieting seems very important to you and you need to do it right, then it is recommended that you visit a professional such as a nutritionist or dietitian to discuss your dieting plan and optimizing it for the better.

No matter how much you want to lose weight, it is not advised that you decrease your calorie intake to an unhealthy level. Losing weight does not mean that you stop eating. It is done by carefully planning meals.

A plant-based diet is very easy once you get into it. At first, you will start to face a lot of difficulties, but if you start slowly, then you can face all the barriers and achieve your goal.

CPSIA information can be obtained
at www.ICGtesting.com
Printed in the USA
BVHW041346190121
598138BV00006B/127

9 781801 592376